Love Your Diet

Calorie Counter

Maximum Calories

The Goldilocks Paradigm

K.J.R. Alexander

Credits

All amounts are extrapolated for different measurements using the standardized US Department of Agriculture Nutrient Database:

http://www.nal.usda.gov/fnic/foodcomp/

USDA National Nutrient Database for Standard Reference Release 22 (2009)

CONTENTS

INTRODUCTION 1

    The Goldilocks Paradigm 1

    How Many Calories Do You Need? 1

    How Much Should You Weigh? 2

        BMI Table 3

        Height Weight Graph 4

        Height Weight Table 5

    Daily Calorie Journal 6

DIET PLAN SUMMARY 6

DAILY MENU MODEL 9

CALORIE COUNTER EXPLANATION 10

CALORIE COUNTER – FOODS TO EAT 11

    Measurements and Abbreviations 12

CALORIE COUNTER – FOODS NOT TO EAT 37
FAST FOODS & LTN FOODS

Introduction

The Love Your Diet *Calorie Counter* is designed to accompany the Love Your Diet books *Light Fantastic* and the *Aphrodite Bread and Wine Diet*. These books explain the diet in detail and reading one of them is necessary for full understanding. *Light Fantastic* is the most inclusive. However, a summary of the diet basics is also included here for reference.

The calorie counter is divided into two parts: calories for the basic good foods to eat on the diet and calories for the foods not to eat – fast foods and the LTN, or Little-To-No foods, as discussed in the books. This helps guide food selection. Following is basic information needed to help guide your diet and count calories.

Maximum Calories: The Goldilocks Paradigm

Not too much and not too little. This is the Goldilocks Paradigm (*pair' a dime*), a pattern or model of thought, used by physicists in the study of the universe. The idea is that everything is balanced and in harmony, as, for example, the stronger and weaker forces in gravity. Not too much and not too little keeps everything just right. Extremes are not the essence. The real essence is somewhere in-between.

Remember, Goldilocks, in the Three Bears' house, checks the chairs, beds, and bowls of porridge belonging to Papa Bear, Mama Bear and Baby Bear. She finds Papa and Mama Bear's too much and too little, but Baby Bear's, for her, are just right! Goldilocks can help! Not too much and not too little, but just right, is a model for the universe. It is also a model to use for your calories for healthy effective dieting.

If you are serious about losing excess weight, the question is not whether you need to count calories. The question is how can you **not** count calories and succeed in the long run. If you don't count calories, you are using someone else's lopsided starvation diet. Calorie counting is the only sane way to mathematically keep track of what you are eating with freedom, choice, and nutrition. Meanwhile, you learn the calorie values of different foods and learn how to read food labels, so necessary in the modern food culture. However, diets that restrict calories to severe limits are not the answer either. Nutritionally unbalanced and severely restricted diets are counterproductive and even dangerous to health. After losing the excess fat, you will not need to count calories.

How Many Calories Do You Need Each Day?

Not too much and not too little, but just right. This is the amount of food you can eat and still lose weight without hunger while following the plan. This is based on the amount of food you are currently eating. Therefore, to count calories for Love Your Diet, you first calculate how many calories you are eating now and set this as your daily upper limit in calories. Some days you will be more hungry and go a little over the target amount. Other days, you will eat less. As you lose weight, your target number for calories also declines. *The effect is that the body naturally relaxes its storage of fat as you replace bad foods with the good foods that are metabolized efficiently.*

How many calories are you now eating to support you current weight? To calculate this amount, simply multiply your current weight by 12, an energy factor selected in Love Your Diet for a sedentary type lifestyle such as sitting at computers or desks and moderate walking. To calculate total calories with the energy factor:

Your current weight x 12 = Your total daily calories.

If you are too hungry, try a 15 factor. The factor is flexible and variable among individuals. What matters is whether you are losing excess fat at the rate of two to five pounds or more per week. This is a real and gentle fat melt and not just water weight as on other diets.

For example, if you weigh 185 pounds, the amount at the 12 factor will be 185 x 12 = 2220 calories, your upper calorie limit for the day. As you eat your own target calories of the good foods guided by the calorie counter, your body automatically reduces fat. Without hunger! As you lose weight, say every five to ten pounds, you will reduce your upper limit in calories. The beauty of this diet is that you will lose weight while eating within 10 pounds of your upper range in calories, *if you are eating the right foods*. You have to severely restrict calories to lose weight *eating the wrong foods*, in turn causing tormenting hunger pains and a body ready to fight back and regain all the fat. Eating good foods but *still eating* the bad foods will also result in no fat loss. The reason is that the good foods can be metabolized and the bad foods "stick to the body" in excess fat. All calories are not equal with today's industrialized foods!

By putting calories per pound with the 12 factor to work for yourself, you can compare each day's calorie intake and weight to see how calories and weight interact. *You can see how your body, when you are eating the natural carbohydrate metabolizer foods, asks with hunger, which you immediately satisfy, for calories just under those required to maintain overweight, with the effect of reducing fat.* If you find you are too hungry, or eating more calories than the amount calculated at the 12 factor, again, you can try a little higher factor, such as 15. The factor is flexible as long as you are losing weight. However, at first, begin the 12 factor as a good starting point.

What Should You Weigh?

Are you overweight? How much do you have to lose to be within a healthy to moderate weight range for your height? Measuring BMI or Body Mass Index is one way to determine where you stand. BMI indicates how much excess fat is on your body. Here is a table that gives height, weight, and BMI. While these amounts are general averages, they are good indicators of healthy weight range. If your weight is not listed due to space limitations, such as 5'8" at 192, which is obese at 197, your category would be in the overweight range bordering on obese. You can also calculate your own BMI online.

Height & Weight in Pounds

BMI	19	20	21	22	23	24	25	26	27	28	29	30	31	32	33	34	35
	Healthy Weight						**Overweight**					**Obese**					
4'10"	91	96	100	105	110	115	119	124	129	134	138	143	148	153	158	162	167
4'11"	94	99	104	109	114	119	124	128	133	138	143	148	153	158	163	168	173
5'	97	102	107	112	118	123	128	133	138	143	148	153	158	163	158	174	179
5'1"	100	106	111	116	122	127	132	137	143	148	153	158	164	169	174	180	185
5'2"	104	109	115	120	126	131	136	142	147	153	158	164	169	175	180	186	191
5'3"	107	113	118	124	130	135	141	146	152	158	163	169	175	180	186	191	197
5'4"	110	116	122	128	134	140	145	151	157	163	169	174	180	186	192	197	204
5'5"	114	120	126	132	138	144	150	156	162	168	174	180	186	192	198	204	210
5'6"	118	124	130	136	142	148	155	161	167	173	179	186	192	198	204	210	216
5'7"	121	127	134	140	146	153	159	166	172	178	185	191	198	204	211	217	223
5'8"	125	131	138	144	151	158	164	171	177	184	190	197	203	210	216	223	230
5'9"	128	135	142	149	155	162	169	176	182	189	196	203	209	216	223	230	236
5'10"	132	139	146	153	160	167	174	181	188	195	202	209	216	222	229	236	243
5'11"	136	143	150	157	165	172	179	186	193	200	208	215	222	229	236	243	250
6'	140	147	154	162	169	177	184	191	199	206	213	221	228	235	242	250	258
6'1"	144	151	159	166	174	182	189	197	204	212	219	227	235	242	250	257	265
6'2"	148	155	163	171	179	186	194	202	210	218	225	233	241	249	256	264	272
6'3"	152	160	168	176	184	192	200	208	216	224	232	240	248	256	264	272	279

Source: Evidence Report of Clinical Guidelines on the Identification, Evaluation, and Treatment of Overweight and Obesity in Adults, 1998. NIH/National Heart, Lung, and Blood Institute (NHLB). Posted at USDA.

Following are two more charts to help you get an idea of how your weight compares.

AVERAGE WEIGHTS AND OVERWEIGHTS FOR MEN AND WOMEN

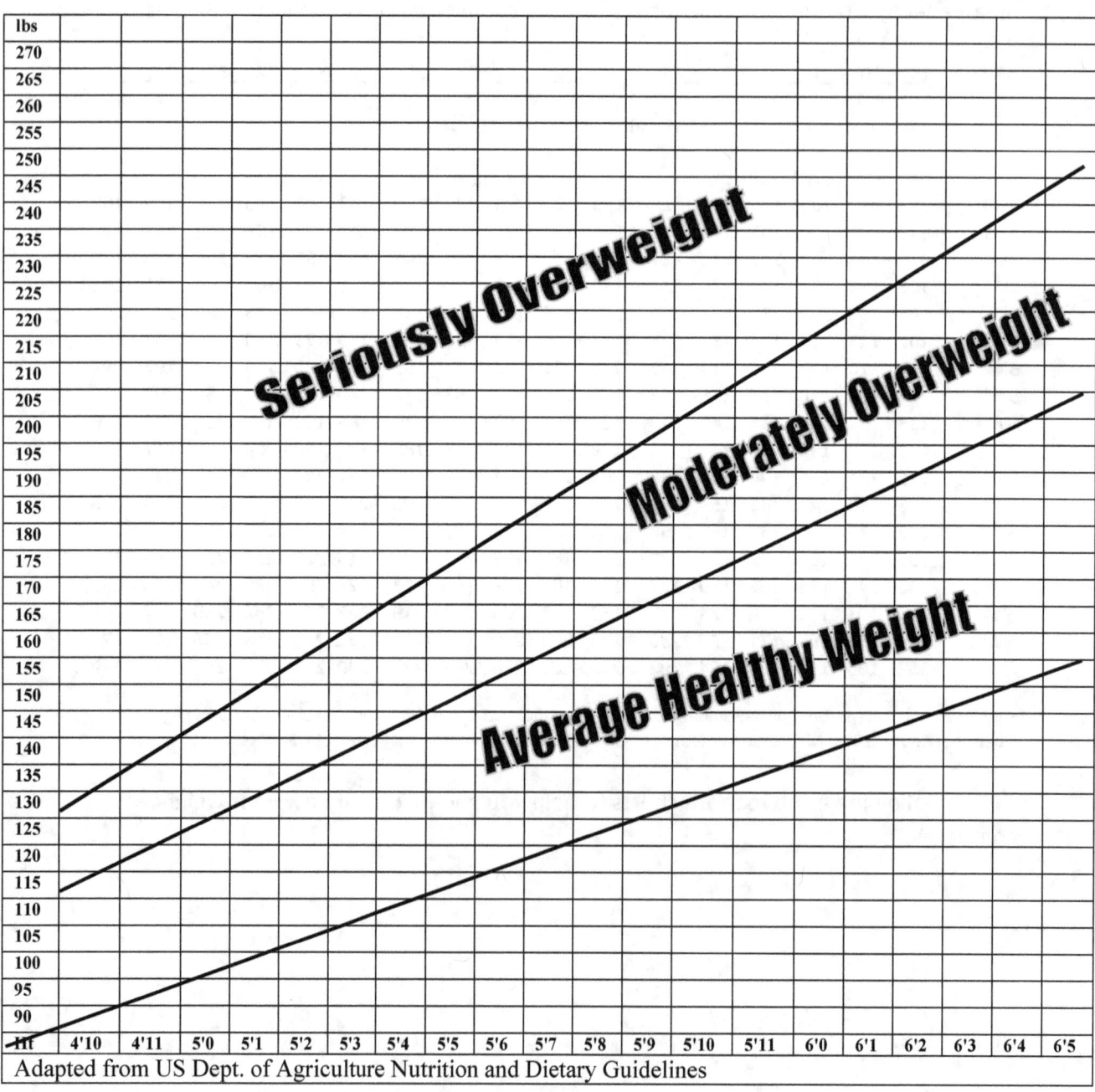

Adapted from US Dept. of Agriculture Nutrition and Dietary Guidelines

Average Healthy Weights for Men and Women by Height and Bone Structure

Women

Average Weights by Height and Bone Structure
without shoes or clothes

	Small	Medium	Large
5'11"	135 to 148	145 to 159	155 to 176
5'10	132 to 145	142 to 156	152 to 172
5'9"	129 to 142	139 to 153	149 to 170
5'8"	126 to 139	136 to 150	146 to 167
5'7"	123 to 136	133 to 147	143 to 163
5'6"	120 to 133	130 to 144	140 to 159
5'5"	117 to 130	127 to 141	137 to 155
5'4"	114 to 127	124 to 138	134 to 151
5'3"	111 to 124	121 to 135	131 to 147
5'2"	108 to 121	118 to 132	128 to 143
5'1"	105 to 118	115 to 129	125 to 140
5'0"	103 to 115	112 to 126	122 to 137
4'11"	101 to 112	110 to 123	119 to 134
4'10"	100 to 110	108 to 120	117 to 131
4'9"	99 to 108	106 to 118	115 to 128

To Determine Bone Structure:

Grasp wrist with opposite hand.
Fingers overlap: Small bone structure
Fingers barely touch: Medium bone structure
Fingers separated: Large bone structure

Men

Average Weights by Height and Bone Structure
without shoes or clothes

	Small	Medium	Large
6'3"	157 to 172	167 to 182	176 to 202
6'2"	153 to 167	163 to 177	171 to 197
6'1"	150 to 163	159 to 173	167 to 192
6'0	147 to 159	155 to 169	163 to 187
5'11"	144 to 155	152 to 165	159 to 183
5'10	141 to 152	149 to 161	156 to 179
5'9"	139 to 149	146 to 158	153 to 175
5'8"	137 to 146	143 to 155	150 to 171
5'7"	135 to 143	140 to 152	147 to 167
5'6"	133 to 140	137 to 149	144 to 163
5'5"	131 to 137	134 to 146	141 to 159
5'4"	129 to 135	132 to 143	139 to 155
5'3"	127 to 133	130 to 140	137 to 151
5'2"	125 to 131	128 to 138	135 to 148
5'1"	123 to 129	126 to 136	133 to 145

Metropolitan Life Insurance Tables, 1983

Weigh Yourself Every Day
Your *Daily Weight and Calorie Journal*

A dieter needs more direction and guidance than just foregoing certain foods in order to stay focused on the diet. The temptation to eat is everywhere in the food environment. It's just too easy to stray once, twice, and thrice, then back to the old eating habits. This is why a *Daily Weight and Calorie Journal* you write yourself is needed. You are able to see the immediate effects of certain foods. You can see on paper the record of what you have eaten and what you weigh each day.

You need to weigh yourself each morning before eating or drinking, without clothes or in the same type clothes each day. You will then list the foods you eat each day and total the calories at the end of the day. You can also write down as many or as few of your thoughts of the day as you wish, your feelings and actions, and what is occurring in your life. You are then more aware of stress and frustration and their possible influences on your eating habits. When you feel good, you can also make note. Your *Daily Weight and Calorie Journal* is a personal part of the adventure into yourself as you lose weight. A piece of paper and pencil will do as will any format you choose, but keep each day's record so you can refer back to it and see progress. For more explanation, see Chapter 8, *Maximum Calories* in Love Your Diet's *Light Fantastic.*

DIET PLAN SUMMARY

Following is a highly-condensed version of Love Your Diet *Light Fantastic.* For more understanding, you need to read the whole book. Love Your Diet is more than calorie counting and is a lot about *how* to choose the right foods. The result is a diet of freedom with lots of choices in foods. However, the following guide is an excellent way to begin to apply your calorie counting.

Stop Starch & Sugar Addiction

If you are overweight, you are eating foods that cause the weight gain. These are manufactured starch and sugar type foods. These foods are addictive and contribute to the constant felt need to eat more and too much. These are the foods on grocery shelves, packaged and full of ingredients that stifle metabolism. It is not enough to only give up foods with gluten, or with corn syrup or sugar, or fat, or certain chemicals, or whatever. These are the foods manufactured for profit rather than for healthy metabolism. To begin the weight loss and to eat comfortably on the diet, you need to give up manufactured, industrialized starch and sugar. Starch and sugar foods are carbohydrate foods. But you do not have to give up carbohydrates. You need only replace the *highly-processed* carbohydrates with *natural* carbohydrates. By following the Love Your Diet *Calorie Counter* as a guide and avoiding the Fast Food Fat and LTN (Little-to-No) Foods, you will be selecting the right foods that are compatible with your natural metabolism. Be sure to eat a variety of foods each day with lots of fruits and vegetables to maintain the balance needed for metabolic energies.

Natural Carbohydrates

You do not have to give up the body's need for carbohydrate foods. You need only to replace the manufactured foods with the natural, real carbohydrates your body can metabolize. This includes a rich cornucopia of lush fruits, vegetables, natural sweets such as honey and raw sugar, and heavy duty natural carbs such as potatoes, rice, beans, and even pasta and bread. This is shown in the calorie counters. Included are the **S** or Sometimes foods and the **LTN** Foods, while losing weight. Bread needs to be all-natural and bakery fresh without added preservatives. See a table of grain products from least to most fattening in *Light Fantastic* or the *Aphrodite Bread and Wine Diet*.

High Protein

Protein is very important to the body. Protein is needed to repair, replace, and build all the cells in the body including muscle, organs, skin, and hair. Adequate protein also helps curb hunger and prevent fatigue while dieting. It also helps maintain skin tone and the skin's ability to "tighten up" and shrink with weight loss. Of the three food categories of carbohydrates, proteins, and fats, protein is the most difficult category to maintain in adequate amounts during dieting. Needed are the foods which supply the EAAs or Essential Amino Acids. (Amino acids are protein.) The body needs daily EAAs in the diet. These are the proteins the body cannot manufacture on its own and must be supplied every day by the diet. To ensure excellent metabolic material, adequate protein is especially needed by the dieter. Foods that contain EAAs, or complete protein are dairy products and meat products such as fish, shellfish, poultry, pork, and beef. Dairy products include milk, yogurt, cottage cheese, and cheese. Eggs also supply complete protein and are very nutritious. Soybean products are the only plant food classified as a complete protein. However, all foods, even fruits and vegetables, have little protein players that contribute to protein synthesis. For this reason, protein amounts are listed in the calorie counters. *For calculating total protein however, you need to count only the EAA foods. These are shown in the last column in the calorie counters with astericks* and show the amount of protein for Column B amounts.*

How much protein do you need each day?

This amount is much higher than most of us eat, especially while dieting. The National Academy of Sciences fixes the amount at half your normal weight. This means your *target* weight, not your overweight. For example, your normal target healthy weight is 160 pounds. This means you should eat half that amount in protein grams or around 80 grams of protein. You may eat more or less than this amount, but this is the target amount. Again, this is calculated using the EAA foods. While dieting, it is especially important to get a good start on the day with a protein breakfast. By contributing to protein needs throughout the day, you are providing adequate metabolic material to burn that excess fat and prevent hunger and fatigue. Love Your Diet structures protein intake throughout the day as shown in the Daily Menu Model.

No Hunger

Maximum Calories
This is described above in the 12 factor calculation and is accomplished using the calorie charts.

Eat When Hungry
Three levels of hunger are identified in *Love Your Diet*.

Hunger Level 1
This is the first twinges of hunger, the signal that you need to eat soon. Level 1 Hunger can be forgotten for small amounts of time.

Hunger Level 2
This is constant feelings of hunger that do not go away. The body signals the need for food.

Hunger Level 3
This is the level of hunger when the body feels it is starving and must have food immediately! Of course, you know it has fat stores to use and is not starving. However this is a survival mechanism by the body. The body is not programmed to endure hunger but interprets Level 3 Hunger as danger of starvation. Willpower can hold up to Level 3 Hunger only so long and then the strongest-willed gives in to the fattest food he or she can find.

On Love Your Diet, Hunger Level 3 is to be avoided! *You are to eat at Level 1 Hunger*. This assures the body that food is available and it is safe to burn excess fat. Again, this is more completely explained in the larger book, Love Your Diet *Light Fantastic* or the *Aphrodite Bread and Wine Diet*, which also include starter menus.

To repeat, as you eat to prevent hunger, but **without highly processed starch and sugar products**, you will see how your body, *on its own*, decreases calorie demand. You immediately feel better and have more energy. The feeling of well-being is so great, you will gladly continue your diet. After all, you are not starving, you are not hungry, and you are replacing empty fat-producing calories with the nutritious food your body appreciates. The body, rather than being signaled to store fat for famine, now feels comfortable with the abundance of nutritious more easily metabolized food such as dairy products, meat, fruits, and vegetables. The body adapts for the "good times" of abundant food supply, close to the land, with good weather and water. Again, this is explained more in the larger book, *Light Fantastic*.

For now, prepare to weigh yourself every morning and count your daily calories determined by the 12 factor calculation. Eat natural, fresh, real foods indicated in the calorie counters. The excess fat will melt away while you are experiencing a satisfying gourmet diet!

DAILY MENU MODEL
Breakfast
15 to 20 grams protein

As dairy is the most compatible with breakfast, this includes milk or dairy products such as yogurt, cottage cheese, and eggs. Kefir is also a highly nutritious filling drink you may want to try if you like buttermilk. You may also use commercial high protein drinks. Read the labels. Include fresh, raw fruit, such as blueberries, apricots, peaches, apples, etc. For lower cholesterol, eat only one egg yolk and add protein with additional whites as for example, 1 whole egg and 2 whites.

Hunger Level 1 Snacks, Morning
8 to 10 grams protein

Hunger level snacks include lowfat dairy foods such as yogurt or cottage cheese and fresh, raw juicy fruit such as cherries and strawberries. High protein drinks may also be used. Eat as much as wanted. Do not choose yogurt packed with extra sugar. Choose the low sugar or artificially sweetened kind around 100 calories. You can also mix all-natural yogurt with no-sugar-added with 1 or 2 tablespoons of the artificially-sweetened and flavored variety, a mixture called LYD or Love Your Diet Yogurt.

Lunch
20+ grams protein

Chicken or fish and raw vegetables and/or raw, fresh fruit.

Hunger Level 1 Snacks, Afternoon
8 to 10 grams protein

Same as morning.

Before Dinner, while preparing food

Raw, fresh vegetables and fruit. Table wine if wanted.

Dinner
20+ grams protein

Meat type food (fish, poultry, beef), heavy duty carb such as potato, rice, or beans, and steamed fresh vegetable with sour cream. Table wine if wanted.

Dessert

Fresh raw fruit with chocolate sauce, honey, raw sugar, no-sugar-added ice cream or cream. Example: banana split with ice cream, chocolate sauce, and peanuts. 70% or more cacao chocolate bar is also good.

After Dinner Hunger Snack

Repeat dessert or choose from nibblers such as nuts, dried fruit, seeds.

Anytime Beverages

These include water, tea, coffee, and moderate intake of diet soda. To flavor tea or coffee, use natural raw sugar or honey and real cream, milk, or half and half and not the artificial creamers. To flavor water, use a tablespoon of all natural, no-sugar-added condensed fruit juice such as cranberry or a fresh lemon.

Again, menus and food lists are available in *Light Fantastic* and the *Aphrodite Bread & Wine Diet*.

Calorie Counters

The two Love Your Diet Calorie Counters are designed for easy use. Here's how to read the calorie counters. The first amount in **Column A**, gives a small portion measure followed in the next column by the calories, which can be multiplied times the amount eaten. Or as an option, the second amount in **Column B** gives the amount of an average serving and the total calories in the following column. The last column is the **Protein Column** showing protein for the measure in Column B. All protein is shown for interest and to indicate all the protein players. As stated earlier, the amount for complete protein foods, Essential Amino Acids or EAAs, are the only proteins to be counted for your daily protein intake and are listed with an asterisk.*

The first part of the calorie counter is the Love Your Diet *Calorie Counter* specifically designed for the diet. The amounts are rounded to the nearest 5 to help daily calculations. This guides food choices that are harmonious to the body's need for nutrition and therefore metabolism. The second part lists calories for *Fast Foods and LTN Foods*, those to avoid while reducing excess fat. These amounts are not rounded to the nearest 5.

Here are the supplies you need for counting calories:

Weight scale for weighing yourself each morning before eating or drinking
Food scale for weighing food in serving sizes in ounces up to at least a pound
Individual measuring cups 2 C, 1 C, ½ C, ¼ C (C= Cup)
1 Tablespoon measure T or tablespoon in the diet
1 teaspoon measure tsp or teaspoon in the diet
Calculator
This Love Your Diet Calorie Counter
Your Daily Weight and Calorie Journal you write

Love Your Diet

Calorie Counter

Measurements and Abbreviations

The following list accompanies your Calorie Counter with explanation of abbreviations and measurements as well as notes about the lists.

---

lb = pound (16 oz)   oz = ounce   C = cup (8 oz)

T = Tablespoon   t or tsp = teaspoon   g = grams

1/4 C = 2 oz   1/2 C = 4 oz   3/4 C = 6 oz   1C = 8 oz

1/ 4 C = 4T   1/2 C = 8T   3/4 C = 12T   1C = 16T   1T = 3 tsp

1 oz = 28.35 grams   3.5 oz = 100 grams   1 lb = 16 oz or 453.6 grams
1 gal = 4 quarts = 3.786 liters = 378 milliliters(ml)   1 quart = 4 C = 2 pints = 946 liter = .946 ml   1C = 30 ml

---

**Please note: The calorie amounts are rounded to the nearest 5 for easier calculation. This accounts for differences in exact Column A and Column B amounts.
Amounts in Fast Foods and LTN Foods are not rounded.**

**Use Calorie Counter amounts to easily calculate calories for servings of different sizes.
Add cooking calories such as cooking oil to cooked food.
Packaged foods: Check labels for calories.
LTN = Little-to-No Intake Foods   S = Sometimes (may be eaten sometimes on diet)
Protein grams are for B serving amounts. Less than .5 gram protein = <.5
EAA, Essential Amino Acid, proteins listed with asterisk.***

Food	Type	A Amt/Calories		B Amt/Calories		Protein Grams EAA*
A						
alfalfa sprouts	raw	**1/2 C**	5	**1 C**	10	1
almonds, see nuts, almonds						
apple	raw, unpeeled	**1 oz**	15	**5 oz**	80	<.5
apple	raw, diced, chopped	**1/4 C**	15	**1 C**	65	<.5
apple butter	spread	**1 T**	30	**2 T**	60	<.5
apple juice, canned or bottled	unsweetened	**1/2 C**	60	**1 C**	120	<.5
applesauce	canned, unsweetened	**1/2 C**	50	**1 C**	105	<.5
apricot	raw	**1 apricot**	20	**1/2C halves**	75	2
apricot, dried	unsweetened, halves	**1/2 C**	155	**1 C**	310	4
artichokes	raw	**1 oz**	15	**1 med**	60	4
artichokes, hearts	cooked	**1/2 C**	40	**1 C**	80	6
asparagus	cooked	**1/2 C**	10	**1 C**	20	4
avocado	peeled, pitted	**1 oz**	45	**7 oz**	315	4
avocado	peeled, sliced	**1/2 C**	115	**1 C**	235	3
B						
bacon, canadian style LTN	cured, cooked	**1 oz**	50	**2 sl**	90	12*
bacon, pork, cured LTN	pan fried	**1 oz**	155	**1 sl**	**45**	3*
bamboo shoots	canned, drained	**1/2 C**	10	**1 C**	25	2
banana	raw	**1 oz**	25	**5 oz**	125	2
bean sprouts, mung	raw	**1/2 C**	15	**1 C**	30	3
bean sprouts, soybean	raw	**1/2 C**	45	**1 C**	90	9
beans, black	cooked	**1/2 C**	115	**1 C**	230	15
beans, garbanzo or chickpeas	cooked	**1/2 C**	140	**1 C**	270	13
beans, great northern	cooked	**1/2 C**	105	**1 C**	210	15

beans, lentils	cooked	**1/2 C**	115	**1 C**	230	18
beans, lima	cooked	**1/2 C**	110	**1 C**	215	15
beans, pea, navy	cooked	**1/2 C**	130	**1 C**	260	15
beans, pinto	cooked	**1/2 C**	125	**1 C**	245	15
beans, red kidney	cooked	**1/2 C**	110	**1 C**	225	15
beans, snap, green, yellow	raw, cooked	**1/2 C**	25	**1 C**	45	2
beans, soy	dry, cooked	**1/2 C**	150	**1 C**	300	29*
Beef						
beef, bottom round, rump roast	cooked, lean only	**1 oz**	55	**4 oz**	220	31*
beef, bottom round, steak	raw, lean only	**1 oz**	45	**4 oz**	180	24*
beef, chuck, arm roast	cooked, lean only	**1 oz**	55	**4 oz**	220	38*
beef, chuck, blade roast	cooked, lean only	**1 oz**	65	**4 oz**	260	35*
beef, corned	cooked	**1 oz**	70	**4 oz**	280	21*
beef, eye of round	raw	**1 oz**	40	**4 oz**	160	25*
beef, eye of round	roasted	**1 oz**	45	**4 oz**	180	33*
beef, flank steak	raw	**1 oz**	40	**4 oz**	160	24*
beef, flank steak	cooked	**1 oz**	55	**4 oz**	220	32*
beef, ground, 75% lean	raw	**1 oz**	80	**4 oz**	320	17*
beef, ground, 75% lean	cooked	**1 oz**	70	**4 oz**	280	27*
beef, ground, 80% lean	raw	**1 oz**	70	**4 oz**	280	19*
beef, ground, 80% lean	cooked	**1 oz**	70	**4 oz**	280	27*
beef, ground, 90% lean	raw	**1 oz**	50	**4 oz**	200	23*
beef, ground, 90% lean	cooked	**1 oz**	60	**4 oz**	240	29*
beef, ground, 95% lean	raw	**1 oz**	40	**4 oz**	160	24*
beef, ground, 95% lean	cooked	**1 oz**	45	**4 oz**	180	29*
beef, heart	raw	**1 oz**	30	**4 oz**	120	19*
beef, kidney	raw	**1 oz**	35	**4 oz**	140	17*
beef, liver	raw	**1 oz**	40	**4 oz**	160	23*

beef, liver	fried	**1 oz**	50	**4 oz**	200	30*
beef, porterhouse steak	raw, 1/4" fat	**1 oz**	65	**4 oz**	260	22*
beef, porterhouse steak	broiled, lean only	**1 oz**	60	**4 oz**	240	31*
beef, rib eye steak	broiled, lean only	**1 oz**	60	**4 oz**	240	30*
beef, rib roast	roasted, lean only	**1 oz**	60	**4 oz**	240	30*
beef, round tip roast	cooked, lean only	**1 oz**	55	**4 oz**	260	31*
beef, round, top round	raw, lean only	**1 oz**	40	**4 oz**	160	26*
beef, round, top round	cooked, lean only	**1 oz**	55	**4 oz**	220	36*
beef, sirloin, top sirloin	raw, lean only	**1 oz**	35	**4 oz**	140	25*
beef, sirloin, top sirloin	cooked, lean only	**1 oz**	50	**4 oz**	200	35*
beef, sirloin, tri tip	raw	**1 oz**	45	**4 oz**	180	23*
beef, sirloin, tri tip	roasted	**1 oz**	60	**4 oz**	240	29*
beef, t bone steak	raw, 1/4" fat	**1 oz**	45	**4 oz**	180	24*
beef, t bone steak	broiled, lean only	**1 oz**	60	**4 oz**	240	31*
beef, tenderloin	raw, 1/8" fat trim	**1 oz**	45	**4 oz**	180	25*
beef, tenderloin	broiled, 1/8" fat trim	**1 oz**	60	**4 oz**	240	33*
beer, 12 oz	regular	**1 oz**	13	**12 oz**	155	2
beer, 12 oz	light	**1 oz**	9	**12 oz**	105	1
beer, 16 oz	regular	**1 oz**	13	**16 oz**	210	2
beer, 16 oz	light	**1 oz**	9	**16 oz**	145	1
beet greens	cooked	**1/2 C**	15	**1 C**	30	4
beets	cooked, slices	**1/2 C**	40	**1 C**	75	3
bison, ground (buffalo)	cooked, patty	**1 oz**	65	**4 oz**	260	27*
black eyed peas	cooked	**1/2 C**	90	**1 C**	180	7
blackberries	raw	**1/2 C**	30	**1 C**	60	2
blueberries	raw	**1/2 C**	40	**1 C**	85	1
bok choy, Chinese cabbage	cooked, sliced	**1/2 C**	10	**1 C**	20	3
boysenberries	frozen, unsweetened	**1 /2 C**	30	**1 C**	60	1

brazil nuts, see nuts						
bread, buns, hamb, hot dog LTN	enriched	**1 avg**	120	**1 avg**	120	3
bread, corn bread S	from recipe 2% milk	**1 oz**	75	**2 oz**	150	4
bread, French or sourdough S	loaf, bakery	**1 oz**	78	**2 oz**	155	5
bread, Indian fry S	Navajo	**1 oz**	94	**2 oz**	188	4
bread, Italian S	enriched, loaf, bakery	**1 oz**	77	**2 oz**	155	5
bread, kneel down S	Navajo	**1 oz**	55	**2 oz**	110	2
bread, mixed grain LTN	sliced, shelf	**1 oz**	70	**26 g sl**	65	3
bread, pita S	4" diameter	**1 oz**	80	**1 4" pita**	80	3
bread, pumpernickel S	loaf	**1 oz**	70	**2 oz**	140	5
bread, raisin LTN	sliced, shelf	**1 oz**	78	**26 g sl**	70	2
bread, rye S	American, sliced	**1 oz**	75	**32 g sl**	85	3
bread, wheat LTN	sliced, shelf	**1 oz**	70	**28 g sl**	70	3
bread, white, enriched LTN	sliced, shelf	**1oz**	75	**25 g sl**	65	2
bread, white, enriched S	homebaked 2% milk	**1 oz**	80	**2 oz**	160	4
bread, white S	homebkd nonfat milk	**1 oz**	78	**2 oz**	160	4
breakfast bars	oats, raisins, coconut	**1 oz**	130	**43 g bar**	200	8
brewers yeast	flakes/supplement	**1 T**	25	**2 T**	50	6*
broccoli	cooked, chopped	**1/2 C**	30	**1 C**	60	4
broccoli	raw, chopped	**1/2 C**	15	**1 C**	30	3
broccoli spear	cooked, 5" long spear	**1 spear**	10	**5" stalk**	50	3
broccoli, flower cluster	raw	**1 floweret**	5	**1 C**	20	2
brussels sprouts	cooked	**1/2 C**	30	**1 C**	60	4
bulgar	cooked	**1/2 C**	75	**1 C**	150	6
butter	spread	**1 tsp**	35	**1 T**	100	<.5*

C

cabbage, Chinese	cooked, sliced	**1/2 C**	10	**1 C**	20	3
cabbage, common varieties	raw, shredded	**1/2 C**	10	**1 C**	20	<1

cabbage, common varieties	cooked	**1/2 C**	15	**1 C**	30	2
cabbage, red	raw, shredded	**1/2 C**	10	**1 C**	20	1
cabbage, savoy	raw, sliced	**1/2 C**	10	**1 C**	20	2
cantaloupe	raw, 5" diam. melon	**1/2 melon**	95	**1 melon**	190	1
cantaloupe	raw, cubes	**1/2 C**	55	**1 C**	110	1
carrot, baby	raw	**1 med**	5	**4 med**	20	<.5
carrots	raw, grated	**1 oz**	12	**1 C**	50	1
carrots	cooked	**1/2 C**	35	**1 C**	70	1
casaba melon	raw	**1/10th avg**	40	**1 melon**	380	2
cashews, see nuts						
catsup	tomato	**1 T**	15	**2 T**	30	<1
cauliflower	raw, floweret	**1**	5	**1 C**	25	2
cauliflower	cooked	**1/2 C**	15	**1 C**	30	2
caviar	red, black	**1 T**	40	**3 T**	120	12*
celery	raw	**1 stalk**	5	**1 C**	20	1
celery	cooked	**1/2 C**	15	**1 C**	30	1
cereal, corn grits, white, yellow	dry, uncooked	**1/4 C**	145	**1/2 C**	290	7
cereal, corn grits, white, yellow	cooked	**1/2 C**	70	**1 C**	145	3
cereal, cream of rice	dry, uncooked	**1/4 C**	160	**1/2 C**	320	5
cereal, cream of rice	cooked	**1/2 C**	65	**1 C**	125	2
cereal, oats, rolled	dry, uncooked	**1/4 C**	75	**1/2 C**	155	6
cereal, oats, rolled	cooked	**1/2 C**	70	**1 C**	145	6
cereal, whole wheat natural	dry, uncooked	**1/4 C**	80	**1/2 C**	160	5
cereal, whole wheat natural	cooked	**1/2 C**	80	**1 C**	160	5
champagne	all	**1 oz**	25	**4 oz**	100	<.5
chard, Swiss	raw or cooked	**1/2 C**	15	**1 C**	25	3
cheese, American	sliced	**1 oz**	105	**2 oz**	210	14*
cheese, average	grated	**1 T**	25	**2 oz**	50	4*

cheese, average	sliced	**1 oz**	100	**2 oz**	200	14*
cheese, brie	sliced	**1 oz**	95	**2 oz**	190	12*
cheese, camembert	sliced	**1 oz**	85	**2 oz**	170	12*
cheese, cheddar	grated	**1 T**	30	**2 T**	60	3*
cheese, cheddar	sliced	**1 oz**	115	**2 oz**	230	14*
cheese, colby	sliced	**1 oz**	110	**2 oz**	220	14*
cheese, cream cheese	spread	**1 oz**	105	**2 oz**	210	4*
cheese, edam	sliced	**1 oz**	100	**2 oz**	200	15*
cheese, feta	sliced	**1 oz**	75	**2 oz**	150	8*
cheese, gouda	sliced	**1 oz**	100	**2 oz**	200	14*
cheese, monterey	sliced	**1 oz**	105	**2 oz**	210	14*
cheese, mozzarella	sliced	**1 oz**	80	**2 oz**	160	12*
cheese, muenster	sliced	**1 oz**	105	**2 oz**	210	14*
cheese, parmesan	grated	**1 T**	25	**2 T**	50	4*
cheese, parmesan	cubed	**1 oz**	110	**1 oz**	110	10*
cheese, provolone	sliced	**1 oz**	100	**2 oz**	200	15*
cheese, Swiss	sliced	**1 oz**	105	**2 oz**	210	15*
cherries	raw, sweet	**1/2 C**	40	**1 C**	80	2

Chicken

Amounts do not include bone weight. Weigh bone after eating and subtract from total weight.

chicken, breast, meat & skin	batter dipped, fried	**1 oz**	75	**4 oz**	300	28*
chicken, breast, meat & skin	flour coated, fried	**1 oz**	65	**4 oz**	260	36*
chicken, breast, meat & skin	fried	**1 oz**	60	**4 oz**	240	36*
chicken, breast, meat & skin	roasted	**1 oz**	55	**4 oz**	220	34*
chicken, breast, meat only	fried	**1 oz**	55	**4 oz**	220	38*
chicken, breast, meat only	roasted	**1 oz**	45	**4 oz**	180	35*
chicken, broiler fryer, meat & skin	batter dipped, fried	**1 oz**	80	**4 oz**	320	26*
chicken, broiler fryer, meat & skin	flour coated, fried	**1 oz**	75	**4 oz**	300	32*

chicken, broiler fryer, meat & skin	roasted	1 oz	70	4 oz	280	31*
chicken, broiler fryer, meat & skin	fried	1 oz	65	4 oz	260	32*
chicken, broiler fryer, meat only	roasted	1 oz	55	4 oz	220	33*
chicken, broiler fryer, meat only	fried	1 oz	60	4 oz	240	34*
chicken, broiler fryer, meat only	stewed	1/2 C	125	1 C	250	31*
chicken, Cornish game hen	roasted, meat & skin	1/2 bird	335	1 whole	670	57*
chicken, Cornish game hen	roasted, meat & skin	1 oz	75	4 oz	300	25*
chicken, drumstick, meat & skin	flour coated, fried	1 oz	70	4 oz	280	31*
chicken, drumstick, meat & skin	fried	1 oz	60	4 oz	240	31*
chicken, drumstick, meat & skin	roasted	1 oz	60	4 oz	240	31*
chicken, drumstick, meat & skin	batter dipped, fried	1 oz	75	4 oz	300	25*
chicken, drumstick, meat only	fried	1 oz	55	4 oz	220	32*
chicken, drumstick, meat only	roasted	1 oz	50	4 oz	200	32*
chicken, giblets	simmered, diced	1/2 C	115	1 C	230	39*
chicken, leg, meat & skin	batter dipped, fried	1 oz	75	4 oz	300	25*
chicken, leg, meat & skin	flour coated, fried	1 oz	70	4 oz	280	30*
chicken, leg, meat & skin	fried	1 oz	65	4 oz	260	30*
chicken, leg, meat & skin	roasted	1 oz	65	4 oz	260	29*
chicken, leg, meat only	fried	1 oz	60	4 oz	240	32*
chicken, leg, meat only	roasted	1 oz	55	4 oz	220	31*
chicken, liver	fried	1 oz	50	4 oz	200	29*
chicken, roasting, meat & skin	roasted	1 oz	65	4 oz	260	27*
chicken, roasting, meat only	roasted	1 oz	50	4 oz	200	28*
chicken, stewing, meat only	stewed, diced	1/2 C	165	1 C	330	43*
chicken, thigh, meat & skin	flour coated, fried	1 oz	75	4 oz	300	30*
chicken, thigh, meat & skin	fried	1 oz	65	4 oz	260	30*
chicken, thigh, meat & skin	roasted	1 oz	70	4 oz	280	28*
chicken, thigh, meat & skin	batter dipped, fried	1 oz	80	4 oz	320	25*

chicken, thigh, meat only	fried	1 oz	65	4 oz	260	31*
chicken, thigh, meat only	roasted	1 oz	60	4 oz	240	30*
chicken, thigh, meat & skin	batter dipped, fried	1 oz	80	4 oz	320	25*
chicken, thigh, meat only	fried	1 oz	65	4 oz	260	31*
chicken, thigh, meat only	roasted	1 oz	60	4 oz	240	30*
chicken, wing, meat & skin	batter dipped, fried	1 oz	90	4 oz	360	23*
chicken, wing, meat & skin	flour coated, fried	1 oz	90	4 oz	360	30*
chicken, wing, meat & skin	fried	1 oz	70	4 oz	280	31*
chicken, wing, meat & skin	roasted	1 oz	80	4 oz	320	30*
chicken, wing, meat only	fried	1 oz	60	4 oz	240	34*
chicken, wing, meat only	roasted	1 oz	60	4 oz	240	34*
chives	raw, chopped	1 T	1	3 T	5	<.5
chocolate fudge topping	thick	1 T	65	2 T	135	2
chocolate syrup topping	thin	1 T	55	2 T	110	1
cocktail sauce, seafood	regular	1 T	10	1/4 C	45	1
coconut	raw	1 oz	100	2 oz	200	2
coconut, flaked	dried, sweetened	1 T	20	1 C	350	2
cod liver oil	supplement/Vit A & D	1 tsp	40	1 T	125	0
coffee	brewed plain	6 oz	2	8 oz	2	<.5
coffee, espresso	brewed plain	1 oz	1	2 oz	1	<.5
coleslaw	home prepared	1/2 C	40	1 C	80	2
collards	raw, chopped	1/2 C	10	1 C	20	2
collards	cooked, chopped	1/2 C	25	1 C	50	4
corn	cooked	1 med ear	75	1 C	130	5
corn grits cereal, white, yellow	dry, uncooked	1/4 C	145	1/2 C	290	7
corn grits cereal, white, yellow	cooked	1/2 C	70	1 C	145	3
cornish game hen	roasted, meat & skin	1/2 bird	335	1 whole	670	57*
cornish game hen	roasted, meat & skin	1 oz	75	4 oz	300	25*

cornmeal, white or yellow	wholegrain	**1 T**	28	**1 C**	440	10
cornmeal, white or yellow	degermed, enriched	**1 T**	32	**1 C**	505	12
cottage cheese, creamed	4% fat small curd	**1/4 C**	55	**1C**	230	28*
cottage cheese, lowfat	1%	**1/4 C**	40	**1C**	165	28*
cottage cheese, lowfat	2%	**1/4 C**	50	**1C**	200	31*
couscous	cooked	**1/2 C**	90	**1 C**	175	6
crab	canned	**1/4 C**	40	**1 C**	160	28*
crab cake	fried	**1 oz**	45	**2 oz**	90	11*
crab, alaska king	steamed	**1 oz**	25	**4 oz**	100	20*
crab, blue	steamed	**1 oz**	30	**4 oz**	120	25*
crab, dungeness	steamed	**1 oz**	30	**4 oz**	120	25*
crabapple	raw	**1 oz**	20	**1 C sl**	85	<.5
cranberries	raw, whole	**1/2 C**	22	**1 C**	45	<.5
cranberries	dried, sweetened	**1/4 C**	90	**1/2 C**	180	<.5
cranberry sauce	canned, sweetened	**1/8 can**	85	**1/2 C**	200	<.5
cream, half and half	fat free	**1 T**	10	**1/4 C**	40	1*
cream, light	coffee or table	**1 T**	30	**1/4 C**	120	3*
cream, nondairy topping	whipped, frozen	**1 T**	15	**1/4 C**	60	0
cream, sour, lowfat	reduced fat	**1 T**	20	**1/4 C**	80	2*
cream, sour, nonfat	nonfat	**1 T**	15	**1/4 C**	45	2*
cream, sour, regular	regular	**1 T**	25	**1/4 C**	100	2*
cream, whipping	light, unwhipped	**1 T**	45	**1/4 C**	180	1*
cream, whipping	heavy, unwhipped	**1 T**	50	**1/4 C**	200	1*
cream, whipping	light, whipped	**1 T**	10	**1/4 C**	90	1*
cream, whipping	heavy, whipped	**1 T**	25	**1/4 C**	100	1*
cream, whipping	pressureized	**1 T**	10	**1/4 C**	40	**<.5**
cream cheese	regular	**1 T**	50	**2 T**	100	2*
cream cheese	regular	**1 oz**	100	**2 oz**	200	4*

cress	raw & cooked	**5 sprigs**	3	**1 C cook**	30	3
cucumber	raw, peeled, sliced	**1/2 C**	5	**1 C**	15	1
currants, black	raw	**1/2 C**	35	**1 C**	70	2
currants, red or white	raw	**1/2 C**	30	**1 C**	65	2
D						
dandelion greens	cooked, chopped	**1/2 C**	20	**1 C**	35	2
dates, deglet noor	whole, pitted	**1**	25	**4**	100	1
dates, medjool	whole.pitted	**1**	65	**2**	130	1
deer, see venison						
dock (sorrel)	raw, chopped	**1/2 C**	15	**1 C**	30	2
duck	roasted, meat only	**1 oz**	60	**1/2 duck**	445	52*
duck, wild, breast	raw, meat only	**1 oz**	35	**1/2 brst**	102	16*
E						
egg	large, whole, fresh	**1**	75	**1**	75	6*
egg white	large	**1**	17	**1**	17	3.6*
egg yolk	large	**1**	55	**1**	55	2.7*
egg, duck	whole, fresh	**1**	130	**1**	130	9*
egg, goose	whole, fresh	**1**	265	**1**	265	20*
egg, lowfat	large	**1**	70	**1**	70	6*
egg, quail	whole, fresh	**1**	14	**2**	28	2*
egg, turkey	whole, fresh	**1**	135	**1**	135	11*
eggplant	raw	**1 C cubed**	20	**1 whole**	130	6
eggplant	cooked	**1/2 C**	15	**1 C**	35	1
elderberries	raw	**1/2 C**	55	**1 C**	105	1
elk, ground	cooked, patty	**1 oz**	55	**4 oz**	110	30*
endive	raw, chopped	**1/2 C**	5	**1 C**	10	<.5

F

figs	raw	**1 med**	40	**2 med**	80	1
figs	dried, uncooked	**1 fig**	20	**2**	50	1
filberts or hazelnuts, see nuts						

Fish (for raw, add any cooking oil amount)

fish fillet, battered or breaded	frozen, heated	**1 fillet**	130	**2 fillets**	260	14*
fish fillet, battered, breaded	fried, fresh	**1 oz**	65	**4 oz**	260	16*
fish stick	breaded, frozen	**1 stick**	70	**4 sticks**	280	12*
fish, anchovy, European	canned in oil	**1 oz**	60	**5 anchov**	40	6*
fish, bass, mixed species	raw	**1 oz**	30	**4 oz**	120	21*
fish, bluefish	raw	**1 oz**	35	**4 oz**	140	23*
fish, burbot	raw	**1 oz**	25	**4 oz**	100	22*
fish, butterfish	raw	**1 oz**	40	**4 oz**	160	20*
fish, carp	raw	**1 oz**	35	**4 oz**	140	20*
fish, catfish, channel	raw, farmed	**1 oz**	40	**4 oz**	160	18*
fish, catfish, channel	raw, wild	**1 oz**	30	**4 oz**	120	19*
fish, cisco	smoked	**1 oz**	50	**2 oz**	100	9*
fish, cod, Atlantic, Pacific	raw	**1 oz**	25	**4 oz**	100	20*
fish, croaker, Atlantic	raw	**1 oz**	30	**4 oz**	120	20*
fish, cusk	raw	**1 oz**	25	**4 oz**	100	22*
fish, dolphin fish	raw	**1 oz**	25	**4 oz**	100	21*
fish, drum	raw, freshwater	**1 oz**	35	**4 oz**	140	20*
fish, eel, mixed species	raw	**1 oz**	50	**4 oz**	200	21*
fish, fish portions	frozen, heated	**1 stick**	70	**2x4x1/2**	140	6*
fish, flatfish, flounder, sole	raw	**1 oz**	25	**4 oz**	100	21*
fish, gefiltefish, commercial	sweet recipe	**1 oz**	25	**1 piece**	35	4*
fish, haddock	raw	**1 oz**	25	**4 oz**	100	21*
fish, halibut, Atlantic, Pacific	raw	**1 oz**	30	**4 oz**	120	24*

fish, herring, Atlantic	raw	**1 oz**	45	**4 oz**	180	20*
fish, herring, Atlantic	kippered	**1 oz**	60	**4 fillets**	17	28*
fish, herring, Atlantic	pickled	**1 oz**	75	**1 piece**	40	2*
fish, herring, Pacific	raw	**1 oz**	55	**4 oz**	220	19*
fish, mackerel, Atlantic	raw	**1 oz**	60	**4 oz**	240	21*
fish, mackerel, Pacific & Jack	raw	**1 oz**	45	**4 oz**	180	23*
fish, mackerel, king	raw	**1 oz**	30	**4 oz**	120	23*
fish, mackerel	canned	**1 oz**	50	**1/2 C**	150	22*
fish, ocean perch	raw	**1 oz**	25	**4 oz**	100	21*
fish, perch, mixed species	raw	**1 oz**	5	**4 oz**	100	22*
fish, pike	raw	**1 oz**	25	**4 oz**	100	22*
fish, pollock, Atlantic	raw	**1 oz**	25	**4 oz**	100	22*
fish, pompano, Florida	raw	**1 oz**	45	**4 oz**	180	21*
fish, rockfish, mixed species	raw	**1 oz**	25	**4 oz**	100	21*
fish, roughy, orange	raw	**1 oz**	20	**4 oz**	80	19*
fish, sable	raw	**1 oz**	55	**2 oz**	110	8*
fish, sable	smoked	**1 oz**	75	**2 oz**	150	10*
fish, salmon, Atlantic	raw, farmed	**1 oz**	50	**4 oz**	200	23*
fish, salmon, coho	raw, wild	**1 oz**	40	**4 oz**	160	24*
fish, salmon, chinook	raw, wild	**1 oz**	50	**4 oz**	200	23*
fish, salmon, pink	canned	**1 oz**	40	**4 oz**	160	22*
fish, salmon, sockeye	canned	**1 oz**	40	**4 oz**	160	23*
fish, salmon	smoked	**1 oz**	60	**4 oz**	240	21*
fish, sardine, Atlantic	canned in oil	**1 small**	25	**1 can**	190	23*
fish, sardine, Pacific	canned/tomato sauce	**1 small**	70	**1 can**	688	77*
fish, sea bass, mixed species	raw	**1 oz**	25	**4 oz**	100	21*
fish, shad, American	raw	**1 oz**	55	**4 oz**	220	19*
fish, shark, mixed species	raw	**1 oz**	35	**4 oz**	140	24*

fish, smelt, rainbow	raw	**1 oz**	25	**4 oz**	100	20*
fish, snapper, mixed species	raw	**1 oz**	30	**4 oz**	120	23*
fish, sturgeon	raw	**1 oz**	30	**4 oz**	120	18*
fish, sole or flounder, flatfish	raw	**1 oz**	25	**4 oz**	100	21*
fish, swordfish	baked or broiled	**1 oz**	35	**4 oz**	140	22*
fish, tilapia	raw	**1 oz**	25	**4 oz**	100	23*
fish, trout, mixed species	raw	**1 oz**	40	**4 oz**	160	24*
fish, trout	raw, farmed	**1 oz**	40	**4 oz**	160	24*
fish, trout	raw, wild	**1 oz**	35	**4 oz**	140	23*
fish, tuna, bluefin	raw	**1 oz**	40	**4 oz**	160	26*
fish, tuna, yellowfin	raw	**1 oz**	30	**4 oz**	120	27*
fish, tuna	canned, water pack	**1 oz**	35	**3 oz**	100	22*
fish, tuna	canned in oil	**1 oz**	55	**3 oz**	170	25*
fish, turbot, European	raw	**1 oz**	25	**4 oz**	100	18*
fish, whitefish, mixed species	raw	**1 oz**	40	**4 oz**	160	22*
fish, whiting	raw	**1 oz**	25	**4 oz**	100	21*
flour, white	enriched, unbleached	**1 T**	28	**1 C**	455	13
flour, whole wheat	whole grain	**1 T**	25	**1 C**	405	16
french fries S	frozen, heated	**1 oz**	50	**10 fries**	125	2
french fries, steak fries S	frozen, heated	**1 oz**	45	**10 fries**	200	3
fudgesicle bars	fat free	**1 oz**	36	**1 pop**	54	3
fudge bar, Klondike Slim A Bear	98% fat free, no sugar	**1 oz**	35	**1 bar**	92	3
fudgesicle pops	no sugar added	**1 oz**	30	**2 pops**	88	3
G						
garlic	raw, cloves	**1 clove**	4	**3**	15	1
garlic	raw, chopped	**1 tsp**	4	**1 T**	15	1
ginger root	fresh, sliced	**1 oz**	15	**1/4 C**	20	<.5
gooseberries	raw	**1/2 C**	30	**1 C**	65	1

grape juice, canned, bottled	unsweetened	**1/2 C**	80	**1 C**	155	1
grapefruit	raw	**1/2 med**	40	**1 med**	80	1
grapefruit juice	canned, unsweetened	**1/2 C**	50	**1 C**	95	1
grapes, seedless	raw	**1/2 C**	55	**1 C**	110	1
grapes, w/seeds	raw	**1/2 C**	50	**1 C**	105	1
green beans, snap, yellow, green	cooked	**1/2 C**	25	**1 C**	45	2
guava	raw, edible portions	**1 fruit**	35	**1 C**	110	4

H

hazelnuts or filberts, see nuts						
honey	raw	**1 tsp**	20	**1 T**	65	<.5
honeydew melon	raw, 6" diameter	**1/4 melon**	115	**1 Ccubes**	60	1
horseradish	prepared	**1 tsp**	2	**1 T**	5	<.5

I

ice cream, chocolate	light, no sugar added	**1/2 C**	110	**1 C**	220	5*
ice cream, chocolate	fat free 98%	**1/2 C**	90	**1 C**	180	5*
ice cream, chocolate LTN	regular	**1/2 C**	145	**1 C**	290	5*
ice cream, chocolate caramel	no sugar added	**1/2 C**	105	**1 C**	215	5*
ice cream, chocolate, frozen milk	fat free	**1/2 C**	115	**1 C**	229	6*
ice cream, french vanilla LTN	softserve regular	**1/2 C**	190	**1 C**	380	7*
ice cream, french vanilla	no sugar added	**1/2 C**	105	**1 C**	210	6*
ice cream, vanilla	light	**1/2 C**	125	**1 C**	250	7*
ice cream, vanilla LTN	regular	**1/2 C**	145	**1 C**	290	5*
ice cream, vanilla	no sugar added	**1/2 C**	100	**1 C**	200	5*
ice cream, vanilla fudge twirl	no sugar added	**1/2 C**	110	**1 C**	220	3*

J

jam	spread	**1 T**	55	**1 T**	55	<.5
jelly	spread	**1 T**	55	**1 T**	55	<.5

K

kale	cooked	1/2 C	20	1 C	35	2
kiwi	raw	1 med	45	2 med	90	2
kohlrabi	cooked, sliced	1/2 C	25	1 C	50	3
kumquat	raw, edible portions	1 med	15	2 med	30	1

L

lamb chop	broiled, lean & fat	1 oz	90	4 oz	360	29*
lamb chop	cooked, lean only	1 oz	60	4 oz	240	34*
lamb shoulder	cooked, lean only	1 oz	60	4 oz	240	28*
lamb, leg	raw	1 oz	65	4 oz	260	20*
lamb, leg	cooked	1 oz	75	4 oz	300	29*
leeks	cooked, bulb & lwr leaf	1/2 C	10	1 C	30	1
lemon	raw	1/2 med	10	1 med	20	<1
lemon juice	raw or canned	1 T	3	1/4 C	15	<.5
lentils, see beans						
lettuce, butterhead, Boston	raw, med leaf	1 leaf	1	1 C	10	1
lettuce, iceburg	raw, med leaf	1 leaf	1	1 C	10	<.5
lettuce, greenleaf	raw, med leaf	1 leaf	1	1 C	5	<.5
lettuce, romaine, cos	raw, med leaf	1 leaf	1	1 C	10	1
lettuce, red leaf	raw, med leaf	1 leaf	1	1 C	5	<.5
lime	raw	1/2 small	10	1 small	20	<.5
lime juice	raw, unsweetened	1 T	5	1/4 C	15	<.5
liquor:gin, vodka, rum, whiskey LTN 80 proof		1 oz	65	1.5 oz	97	0
liquor:gin, vodka, rum, whiskey LTN 86 proof		1 oz	70	1.5 oz	105	0
liquor:gin, vodka, rum, whiskey LTN 90 proof		1 oz	73	1.5 oz	110	0
lobster	steamed	1 oz	40	5 oz	200	30*
loganberries	frozen, thawed	1/2 C	40	1 C	80	2

M

macadamia nuts, see nuts

macaroni S	cooked	**1/2 C**	110	**1 C**	220	8
mango	raw, 8 oz	**1 mango**	135	**1 C sl**	105	1
maple syrup	natural	**1 T**	50	**1/4 C**	200	0
margarine	spread	**1 tsp**	35	**1 T**	100	<.5
mayonnaise	fat free	**1 tsp**	5	**1 T**	15	<.5
mayonnaise	light	**1 tsp**	15	**1 T**	50	<.5
mayonnaise	regular	**1 tsp**	35	**1 T**	100	<.5
meatless burger	mix, dry	**1/2 C**	115	**1 C**	230	22*
milk, instant, nonfat	dry	**1 T**	15	**1/3 C**	80	8*
milk, lowfat	1% fat	**1/2 C**	50	**1C**	100	8*
milk, reduced fat	2% fat	**1/2 C**	60	**1C**	120	8*
milk, skim	nonfat	**1/2 C**	45	**1C**	85	8*
milk, whole	3.25% fat	**1/2 C**	70	**1C**	145	8*
molasses	light	**1 T**	50	**1/4 C**	200	0
molasses, blackstrap	dark, unrefined	**1 T**	45	**1/4 C**	180	0
mushrooms	raw, sliced	**1/2 C**	10	**1 C**	20	2
mushrooms	cooked	**1/2 C**	20	**1 C**	40	3
mushrooms, shitake	cooked	**1/2 C**	40	**1 C**	80	2
mushrooms, shitake	dried	**1**	10	**2**	20	1
mustard	yellow	**1 tsp**	3	**1 T**	10	1
mustard greens	cooked, chopped	**1/2 C**	10	**1 C**	20	3

N

nectarine	raw, 5 oz	**1 oz**	15	**5 oz**	75	2
noodles, chow mein S	cooked	**1/2 C**	120	**1 C**	235	4
noodles, egg S	cooked	**1/2 C**	110	**1 C**	220	7
noodles, egg, spinach S	cooked	**1/2 C**	105	**1 C**	210	8

nuts, almonds	raw, whole	**1 T**	50	**1 C**	827	30
nuts, almonds	raw, slivered	**1 T**	40	**1 C**	624	23
nuts, almonds	raw, sliced	**1 T**	35	**1 C**	532	20
nuts, brazil nuts	raw, whole	**1 T**	55	**1 C**	918	20
nuts, cashews	dry, oil rstd, w/o salt	**1 T**	50	**1 C**	786	21
nuts, filberts or hazelnuts	raw, chopped	**1 T**	45	**1 C**	722	17
nuts, filberts or hazelnuts	raw, whole	**1 T**	55	**1 C**	848	20
nuts, macadamia	raw	**1 T**	60	**1 C**	962	11
nuts, mixed	dry roasted, w/o salt	**1 T**	50	**1 C**	814	24
nuts, peanuts	dry roasted, w/o salt	**1 T**	55	**1 C**	854	35
nuts, peanuts, spanish	oil roasted, w/o salt	**1 T**	55	**1 C**	851	41
nuts, pecans	raw, halves	**1 T**	40	**1 C**	684	9
nuts, pecans	raw, chopped	**1 T**	45	**1 C**	753	10
nuts, pine nuts	dried	**1 T**	55	**1 C**	909	18
nuts, pistachios	raw	**1 T**	40	**1 C**	685	25
nuts, walnuts, black	dried, chopped	**1 T**	50	**1 C**	772	30
nuts, walnuts, English	raw, halves	**1 T**	40	**1 C**	654	15
nuts, walnuts, English	raw, chopped	**1 T**	45	**1 C**	765	18

O

oatmeal, regular	dry, uncooked	**1/4 C**	75	**1/2 C**	155	6
oatmeal, regular	cooked	**1/2 C**	70	**1 C**	145	6
oils, salad, cooking, vegetable	olive, canola, etc.	**1 T**	120	**1 T**	120	<.5
okra	cooked	**1/2 C**	25	**1 C**	50	3
olives, black	canned, black	**1 lrg**	5	**10 lrg**	50	1
olives, green	canned, green, pickled	**1 med**	4	**10**	40	1
onions	raw, chopped	**1 T**	5	**1/2 C**	35	1
onions	raw	**1 slice**	5	**1 med**	45	1
onions	chopped, sautéed	**1/2 C**	60	**1 C**	115	1

onions	dehydrated flakes	**1 tsp**	5	**1 T**	20	<.5
onions, green	raw, bulb and tops	**1 whole**	5	**1/2 C**	15	1
orange	raw	**1 oz**	15	**4 oz**	60	1
orange juice	raw	**1/2 C**	55	**1 C**	110	2
orange juice	canned, unsweetened	**1/2 C**	50	**1 C**	105	1
orange juice	from frozen concentrate	**1/2 C**	55	**1 C**	110	2
oyster, Pacific	raw	**1 med**	40	**4 med**	160	5*
oyster, eastern	raw, wild	**1 med**	10	**6 med**	60	6*
oyster, eastern	raw, farmed	**1 med**	7	**6 med**	50	4*
oyster, eastern	breaded, fried	**1 med**	30	**6 med**	175	7*

P

pancakes S	plain, 4" diameter	**1**	85	**2**	170	6
pancakes S	whole wheat, 4" diam	**1**	90	**2**	180	8
papaya	raw, edible portion	**1 oz**	10	**1 med**	120	2
parsley	raw, sprigs	**1 T**	1	**10**	4	<.5
parsnips	cooked	**1 oz**	20	**1 C**	110	1
passion fruit (granadilla)	raw, edible portion	**1 oz**	25	**1 fruit**	20	<.5
pasta, various S	cooked	**1/2 C**	100	**1 C**	200	8
peach	raw	**1 oz**	10	**4 oz**	40	1
peach	dried, halves	**1 half**	30	**3**	95	1
peach	canned, juice pack	**1 half**	45	**1 C**	110	2
peanut butter	reg, smooth or chunky	**1 T**	95	**2 T**	190	8
peanuts, see nuts						
pear	raw	**1 oz**	17	**7 oz**	120	1
pear	canned, juice pack	**1 half**	40	**1 C**	125	1
peas	raw	**1/2 C**	60	**1 C**	120	9
peas	canned or frozen	**1/2 C**	60	**1 C**	120	8
peas, edible pod	cooked	**1/2 C**	35	**1 C**	70	5

peas, split, dry	cooked	**1/2 C**	115	**1 C**	230	16
pecans, see nuts						
peppers, hot chili, green, red	raw	**1**	20	**1/2 C**	30	1
peppers, sweet, green, red, yellow	raw	**1 oz**	7	**6 oz**	40	2
pickle relish	sweet	**1 tsp**	7	**1 T**	20	<.5
pickles	dill	**1 slice**	1	**4 slices**	5	1
pickles	sweet (gherkins)	**1 midget**	10	**1/4 C sl**	50	<.5
pickles	sour, slices	**1 slice**	1	**1/4 C**	5	<.5
pimientos	canned	**1 T**	3	**1 med**	15	1
pine nuts, see nuts						
pineapple	raw, diced	**1 oz**	15	**1 C**	75	1
pineapple juice	canned, unsweetened	**1/2 C**	65	**1 C**	130	1
pistachios, see nuts						
pizza, cheese S	12" diameter	**2" slice**	185	**4" sl**	370	varies
pizza, meat/vegetables S	12" diameter	**2" slice**	245	**4" sl**	490	varies
pizza, pepperoni LTN	12" diameter	**2" slice**	240	**4" sl**	480	varies
plums	raw	**1 oz**	15	**2 oz**	30	<.5
pomegranate	raw	**1/2 pom**	50	**1 pom**	105	1
popcorn	plain, air popped	**1 C**	30	**2 C**	60	2
popcorn	popped w/oil, salted	**1 C**	55	**2 C**	110	2
pork, bacon LTN	pan fried	**1 oz**	150	**1 slice**	40	3*
pork, bacon, Canadian style LTN	unheated	**1 oz**	45	**2 sl**	90	12*
pork, bacon, Canadian style LTN	cooked	**1 oz**	50	**2 sl**	90	12*
pork, chop	pan broiled, lean	**1 oz**	50	**4 oz**	200	33*

pork, ham (All ham is LTN due to processing and curing, but some lean may be tolerated.)

pork, ham	cured, roasted, lean	**1 oz**	60	**4 oz**	240	35*
pork, ham	cured, rstd, lean & fat	**1 oz**	75	**4 oz**	310	31*
pork, ham, extra lean	cured, roasted	**1 oz**	40	**4 oz**	160	24*

pork, ham, extra lean	cured, unheated	**1 oz**	35	**4 oz**	140	22*
pork, ham, extra lean & regular	cured, unheated	**1 oz**	45	**4 oz**	180	21*
pork, ham, lean & fat	cured, unheated	**1 oz**	70	**4 oz**	280	21*
pork, ham, rump half	fresh, roasted, lean	**1 oz**	60	**4 oz**	240	35*
pork, ham, shank half	fresh, roasted, lean	**1 oz**	60	**4 oz**	240	32*
pork, ham, whole	cured, unheated	**1 oz**	40	**4 oz**	160	25*
pork, ham, whole, lean only	cured, roasted	**1 oz**	45	**4 oz**	180	28*
pork, loin roast	cooked, lean only	**1 oz**	65	**4 oz**	260	31*
pork, ribs, country style	cooked, lean & fat	**1 oz**	85	**4 oz**	340	27*
pork, ribs, country style	cooked, lean only	**1 oz**	65	**4 oz**	260	30*
pork, sausage, ground LTN	patty, cooked	**1 oz**	100	**2 oz**	200	10*
pork, sausage, link LTN	cooked	**1 link**	80	**2 links**	160	14*
pork, shoulder, roast	cooked, lean	**1 oz**	65	**4 oz**	260	27*
pork, shoulder, steak	cooked, lean	**1 oz**	90	**4 oz**	320	33*
pork, spareribs	cooked, lean & fat	**1 oz**	110	**4 oz**	440	33*
pork, tenderloin	cooked, lean	**1 oz**	55	**4 oz**	220	34*
potato	baked, flesh only	**1 oz**	26	**10 oz**	260	6
potato	raw, diced or sliced	**1/2 C**	60	**1 C**	120	3
potato	mashed w/milk & butter	**1/2 C**	110	**1 C**	220	4
potato	boiled, peeled	**1/2 C**	65	**1 C**	135	3
potato, french fries, fast food LTN	french fries	**1 oz**	100	**3 oz**	300	2
potato, wedges	from frozen	**1 oz**	35	**10 oz**	350	6
potato chips LTN	plain	**1 oz**	150	**6 oz**	900	12
prune juice	canned	**1/2 C**	90	**1 C**	180	2
prunes	dried	**1 prune**	20	**5**	100	1
pudding, instant, dry (add milk)	fat free, sugar free	**1 oz**	95	**8 g pkt**	25	<.5
pudding, instant, chocolate	prepared w/2% milk	**1/2 C**	155	**1 C**	310	9*
pumpkin	canned	**1/2 C**	40	**1 C**	85	3

pumpkin and squash seed kernels	dried	**1 T**	45	**1 C**	720	39
pumpkin and squash seed kernels	roasted, w/o salt	**1 T**	42	**1 C**	680	35
pumpkin and squash seeds	whole, rstd, w/o salt	**1 T**	20	**1 C**	285	12
Q, R						
radish	raw	**1 radish**	1	**10**	10	<.5
raisins	seedless	**1 T**	30	**1/4 C**	120	1
raspberries	raw	**1/2 C**	30	**1 C**	65	2
raspberries	frozen, sweetened	**1 T**	15	**1/4 C**	85	<.5
rice, brown, medium/long grain	cooked	**1/2 C**	105	**1 C**	215	4
rice, white, long grain	cooked	**1/2 C**	100	**1 C**	205	4
rice, white, short/medium grain	cooked	**1/2 C**	120	**1 C**	210	4
rice, wild	cooked	**1/4 C**	40	**1/2 C**	80	3
rice cakes, brown rice	plain	**1 oz**	110	**1 cake**	35	1
rice cakes, brown rice	sesame seed	**1 oz**	111	**1 cake**	35	1
rutabaga	cooked, diced	**1/2 C**	30	**1 C**	65	2
S						
salad dressings	lowfat	**1 T**	20	**1 T**	20	<.5
salad dressings	regular	**1 T**	70	**1 T**	70	<.5
salsa	ready to serve	**1 T**	5	**1/4 C**	20	<.5
sauerkraut	canned, undrained	**1/2 C**	20	**1 C**	45	2
scallop	raw	**1 oz**	25	**4 oz**	100	20*
scallop	breaded, fried	**1 oz**	60	**2 lrg**	70	6*
sesame seeds	whole, dried	**1 T**	50	**1 C**	825	26
shallots	raw, chopped	**1 T**	7	**1/4 C**	30	1
shrimp	fresh	**1 oz**	30	**4 lrg**	30	6*
shrimp	breaded, fried	**1 oz**	70	**3 oz**	210	18*
shrimp	breaded, fried	**1 large**	75	**6 lrg**	450	38*
soda pop, regular LTN	cola, root beer, etc	**1 oz**	12	**12 oz**	135-180	0

soda pop, diet	cola, root beer, etc	**1 oz**	0	**12 oz**	0 - 5	0
soda, club	carbonated, plain	**1 oz**	0	**12 oz**	0	0
sour cream	reduced fat, cultured	**1 T**	20	**1/4 C**	80	2*
sour cream	nonfat	**1 T**	10	**1/4 C**	40	2*
sour cream	regular	**1 T**	25	**1/4 C**	100	3*
soy burger	mix, dry	**1/2 C**	115	**1 C**	230	22*
soy sauce and tamari	regular	**1 tsp**	3	**1 T**	10	1
spaghetti S	enriched, cooked	**1/2 C**	110	**1 C**	220	8
spaghetti, spinach S	cooked	**1/2 C**	90	**1 C**	180	6
spaghetti, whole wheat S	cooked	**1/2 C**	85	**1 C**	175	7
spaghetti sauce	ready to serve	**1/2 C**	90	**1 C**	185	5
spinach	raw	**1 leaf**	2	**1 C**	10	1
spinach	cooked	**1/2 C**	20	**1 C**	40	5
squash, summer, all varieties	cooked, sliced	**1/2 C**	20	**1 C**	35	2
squash, winter, all varieties	cooked, baked	**1/2 C**	40	**1 C**	75	2
strawberries	raw, sliced	**1/2 C**	25	**1 C**	50	1
strawberries	frozen, unsweetened	**1/4 C**	25	**1/2 C**	50	1
submarine sandwich S	tuna salad w/mayo	**1 oz**	65	**8 oz**	585	30*
submarine sandwich S	turkey, ham, vegetables	**1 oz**	55	**8 oz**	456	22*
submarine sandwich S	roast beef	**1 oz**	55	**8 oz**	410	29*
sugar, brown	refined	**1 tsp**	10	**1 T**	35	0
sugar, raw brown	unrefined	**1 tsp**	5	**1 T**	15	<.5
sugar, white granulated LTN	beet or cane, refined	**1 tsp**	15	**1 T**	45	0
sunflower seed kernels	dried	**1 T**	50	**1 C**	821	33
sunflower seed kernels	dry roasted, w/o salt	**1 T**	45	**1 C**	745	25
sunflower seeds w/hulls	dried	**1 T**	15	**1 C**	262	10
sweet potato	baked, boiled	**1 oz**	25	**10 oz**	250	6
Swiss chard	cooked, chopped	**1/2 C**	15	**1 C**	35	3

syrup, maple	natural maple	**1 T**	50	**1/4 C**	200	0
T						
tangerine	raw	**1 oz**	15	**4 oz**	60	1
tea	black, herb	**1 oz**	0	**1 C**	2	0
tofu	firm	**1 oz**	20	**2 oz**	40	4*
tofu	soft	**1 oz**	15	**2 oz**	30	4*
tomato	raw	**1/4" sl**	5	**1 C**	30	2
tomato	stewed	**1/2 C**	40	**1 C**	80	2
tomato juice	canned	**1/2 C**	20	**1 C**	40	2
tomato paste	canned	**1/2 C**	105	**6 oz can**	140	7
tomato puree	canned	**1/2 C**	50	**1 C**	100	4
tomato sauce	canned	**1/2 C**	40	**1 C**	80	3
tomato, chopped or sliced	raw	**1/2 C**	15	**1 C**	30	2
tortilla, yellow corn S	6" diameter	**1**	60	**2**	180	2
tortilla, flour S	7 to 8" diameter	**1**	145	**2**	290	8
turkey, dark meat	roasted, meat only	**1 oz**	55	**4 oz**	220	32*
turkey, light meat	roasted, meat only	**1 oz**	45	**4 oz**	180	34*
turnip	cooked, cubes	**1/2 C**	15	**1 C**	35	1
turnip greens	cooked	**1/2 C**	15	**1 C**	30	2
U, V, W						
vegetable juice	canned	**1/2 C**	25	**1 C**	45	1
vegetable stew meatless	homemade	**1 C**	60	**2 C**	120	4
vegi burger	cooked	**1 oz**	30	**3 oz**	90	14*
vinegar	cider, distilled	**1 T**	2	**1/4 C**	10	0
venison	cooked	**1 oz**	45	**4 oz**	180	34*
venison, ground	cooked, patty	**1 oz**	55	**4 oz**	110	30*
venison, loin steak	cooked	**1 oz**	45	**4 oz**	180	34*
walnuts, see nuts						

water chestnuts, Chinese	canned	**4 avg**	15	**1 C sl**	35	1
watercress	raw, sprigs	**10**	3	**1 C**	5	1
watermelon	raw, cubed	**1 oz**	10	**1 C**	45	1
wheat bran	raw	**1 T**	8	**1 C**	120	9
wheat germ	raw	**1 T**	25	**2 T**	50	4
wheat germ oil	supplement/Vit E	**1 tsp**	40	**1 T**	125	<.5
whipped topping	frozen	**1 T**	15	**1/4 C**	60	0
whipped topping, light	frozen	**1 T**	10	**1/4 C**	40	0
whole wheat natural cereal	dry, uncooked	**1/4 C**	80	**1/2 C**	160	5
whole wheat natural cereal	cooked	**1/2 C**	160	**1 C**	160	5
wine, dessert	sweet	**1 oz**	45	**4 oz**	180	<.5
wine, table	red, white	**1 oz**	25	**6 oz**	150	<.5

X, Y, Z

yams	baked, boiled	**1 oz**	35	**10 oz**	350	4
yogurt butter	oil/yogurt spread	**1 tsp**	15	**1 T**	45	0
yogurt, frozen, soft serve LTN	choc, vanilla	**1/2 C**	115	**1 C**	230	6*
yogurt, frozen, chocolate, nonfat	no sugar added	**1/2 C**	100	**1 C**	199	8*
yogurt, lowfat	artificial sweetener	**1 oz**	14	**8 oz**	110	8*
yogurt, lowfat LTN	sugar, fruit ,flavorings	**1 oz**	29	**8 oz**	240	11*
yogurt, lowfat	all natural, plain	**1 oz**	19	**8 oz**	150	11*
yogurt, lowfat plus milk solids	plain	**1 oz**	18	**8 oz**	145	12*
yogurt, nonfat	artificial sweetener	**1 oz**	13	**8 oz**	100	9*
yogurt, nonfat	plain	**1 oz**	16	**8 oz**	130	13*
yogurt, nonfat LTN	sugar, fruit, flavorings	**1 oz**	27	**8 oz**	215	10*
yogurt, whole	plain	**1 oz**	18	**8 oz**	140	8*

Love Your Diet

Fast Foods & LTN Foods

Calorie Counter

Food	A Amt	Calories	B Amt	Calories	B Protein grams EAA*
A B					
biscuit, scone	**1 oz**	100	**3 oz**	300	4
biscuit, w/bacon, egg, & cheese, McDonald's	**1 oz**	86	**1**	441	19*
biscuit, w/egg	**1 oz**	78	**1**	373	12*
biscuit, w/egg & bacon	**1 oz**	86	**1**	458	17*
biscuit, w/egg & ham	**1 oz**	68	**1**	461	20*
biscuit, w/egg & sausage	**1 oz**	92	**1**	581	19*
biscuit, w/egg & steak	**1 oz**	79	**1**	410	18*
biscuit, w/ham	**1 oz**	97	**1**	386	13*
biscuit, w/sausage	**1 oz**	111	**1**	485	12*
bologna, beef	**1 oz**	89	**28g sl**	88	3*
bologna, beef & pork	**1 oz**	87	**1 oz sl**	87	4*
bologna, beef & pork, low fat	**1 oz**	65	**28g sl**	64	3*
bologna, chicken, pork	**1 oz**	95	**28g sl**	94	3*
bologna, chicken, pork, beef	**1 oz**	77	**28g sl**	76	3*
bologna, pork	**1 oz**	70	**28g sl**	69	4*
bologna, turkey	**1 oz**	59	**28g sl**	59	3*
bread, mixed grain, shelf, sliced	**1 oz**	71	**26g sl**	65	3
bread, white, shelf, sliced	**1 oz**	75	**25g sl**	66	2
bread, whole wheat, shelf, sliced	**1 oz**	70	**28g sl**	69	3
Breakfast, McDonald's Big	**1 oz**	78	**1**	732	28*
Breakfast, McDonald's Deluxe	**1 oz**	79	**1**	1219	33*
Burrito Supreme, w/beef, Taco Bell	**1 oz**	54	**1**	469	20*
Burrito Supreme, w/chicken, Taco Bell	**1 oz**	51	**1**	444	24*
Burrito Supreme, w/steak, Taco Bell	**1 oz**	52	**1**	454	23*

burrito, bean, Taco Bell	**1 oz**	58	**1**	404	16
burrito, w/beans	**1 oz**	58	**2 pieces**	447	14
burrito, w/beans & cheese	**1 oz**	58	**2 pieces**	378	15*
burrito, w/beans, cheese, & beef	**1 oz**	46	**2 pieces**	331	15*
burrito, w/beef	**1 oz**	67	**2 pieces**	524	27*

C

cake, angel food	**1 oz**	73	**3 oz**	219	5
cake, boston cream pie	**1 oz**	71	**1/6 pie**	232	2
cake, brownie	**1 oz**	132	**2" sq**	112	2
cake, chocolate w/frosting	**1 oz**	104	**1/8 cake**	235	3
cake, fruitcake	**1 oz**	92	**2 oz**	185	2
cake, gingerbread	**1 oz**	101	**1/9 piece**	263	3
cake, pineapple upside-down	**1 oz**	90	**4 oz**	367	4
cake, pound prepared w/butter	**1 oz**	110	**2 oz**	232	3
cake, snack cake, sponge, crème-filled	**1 oz**	103	**1 cake**	157	1
cake, snack cupcakes, choc w/frosting, crème-filled	**1 oz**	107	**1 ccake**	188	2
cake, sponge	**1 oz**	82	**2 oz**	164	3
cake, white, w/coconut frosting	**1 oz**	101	**2 oz**	202	2
cake, yellow, w/vanilla frosting	**1 oz**	106	**2 oz**	112	2
candy, 5th Avenue candy bar	**1 oz**	137	**2 oz**	270	5
candy, Almond Joy	**1 oz**	136	**1.8g pkg**	235	2
candy, average	**1 oz**	135	**2 oz**	270	2
candy, Caramello candy bar	**1 oz**	131	**1.6 oz bar**	208	3
candy, fudge, chocolate w/nuts, from recipe	**1 oz**	131	**2 oz**	262	2
candy, fudge, chocolate, prepared from recipe	**1 oz**	117	**2 oz**	234	1
candy, fudge, vanilla, prepared from recipe	**1 oz**	109	**2 oz**	218	<1
candy, M&M Mars, TWIX choc fudge cookie bars	**1 oz**	156	**2 oz bar**	312	4

candy, milk chocolate bar	**1 oz**	152	**1.5 oz bar**	235	2
candy, Milky Way candy bar	**1 oz**	124	**3.6 oz bar**	450	2
candy, Mounds	**1 oz**	138	**1.9 oz bar**	258	2
candy, Reese's Peanut Butter Cups	**1 oz**	146	**2 cups**	232	3
cereal, bran flakes	**1 oz**	91	**1 C**	128	4
cereal, composite character (movies, TV)	**1 oz**	110	**1 C**		
cereal, corn flakes	**1 oz**	102	**1 C**	101	2
cereal, corn grits, instant, dry	**1 oz**	97	**1 pkt**	96	2
cereal, General Mills Cheerios	**1 oz**	105	**1 C**	111	4
cereal, General Mills Frosted Cheerios	**1 oz**	108	**1 C**	115	2
cereal, General Mills Lucky Charms	**1 oz**	108	**1 C**	114	2
cereal, General Mills Wheat Chex	**1 oz**	98	**1 C**	104	3
cereal, General Mills Wheaties	**1 oz**	101	**1 C**	106	3
cereal, Kellogg's Cocoa Krispies	**1 oz**	108	**1 C**	157	2
cereal, Kellogg's Frosted Flakes	**1 oz**	104	**1 C**	152	1
cereal, Kellogg's Frosted Flakes, 1/3 less sugar	**1 oz**	107	**1 C**	117	2
cereal, Kellogg's Product 19	**1 oz**	94	**1 C**	100	2
cereal, Kellogg's Rice Krispies	**1 oz**	110	**1 C**	108	2
cereal, Kellogg's Special K	**1 oz**	107	**1 C**	117	7
cereal, Kraft, Post, corn flakes, Post Toasties	**1 oz**	102	**1 C**	101	2
cereal, Kraft, Post, frosted shredded wht, bite-size,	**1 oz**	100	**1 C**	183	4
cereal, Kraft, Post, Marshmallow Alpha-bits	**1 oz**	113	**1 C**	115	2
cereal, Kraft, Post, Raisin Bran	**1 oz**	90	**1 C**	178	5
cereal, Kraft, Post, shredded wheat, spoon size	**1 oz**	96	**1 C**	167	5
cereal, oats, instant, fortified, plain, dry	**1 oz**	105	**1 pkt**	103	4
cereal, puffed rice	**1 oz**	109	**1 C**	54	1
cereal, puffed wheat	**1 oz**	104	**1 C**	44	2

cereal, Quaker Cap'n Crunch	**1 oz**	114	**1 C**	144	2
cereal, Quaker Oats and Honey	**1 oz**	129	**1/2 C**	232	5
cereal, Quaker Oats Life	**1 oz**	106	**1 C**	160	4
cereal, Ralston Crispy Rice	**1 oz**	103	**1 C**	102	2
cereal, shredded wheat, plain, biscuit	**1**	84	**2**	155	5
cheeseburger, Burger King	**1 oz**	81	**1**	380	19*
cheeseburger, large, double patty, w/cond & veg	**1 oz**	77	**1**	704	38*
cheeseburger, large, single patty, w/bacon & cond	**1 oz**	88	**1**	608	32*
cheeseburger, large, single patty, w/cond & veg.	**1 oz**	73	**1**	563	28*
cheeseburger, McDonald's	**1 oz**	75	**1**	313	15*
cheeseburger, McDonald's double	**1 oz**	75	**1**	458	26*
cheeseburger, regular, double patty w/cond & veg	**1 oz**	71	**1**	417	21*
cheeseburger, triple patty, plain	**1 oz**	74	**1**	796	56*
cheeseburger, Wendy's Classic Single w/cheese	**1 oz**	63	**1**	522	35*
chicken, boneless, breaded, fried	**1 oz**	84	**6 pieces**	285	15*
chicken, breaded, fried, dark meat	**1 oz**	82	**2 pieces**	431	30*
chicken, breaded, fried, light meat	**1 oz**	86	**2 pieces**	494	36*
chicken, Burger King Chicken Tenders	**1 oz**	82	**6 pieces**	266	13*
chicken, Burger King Chicken Whopper sandwich	**1 oz**	61	**1**	588	32*
chicken, Burger King Original Chicken sandwich	**1 oz**	81	**1**	583	31*
chicken, fillet sandwich	**1 oz**	80	**1**	515	24*
chicken, fillet sandwich w/cheese	**1 oz**	79	**1**	632	29*
chicken, McDonald's Caesar Salad w/crispy chicken	**1 oz**	27	**1 salad**	294	25*
chicken, McDonald's Chicken McGrill w/mayo	**1 oz**	54	**1**	405	28*
chicken, McDonald's Chicken McGrill w/o mayo	**1 oz**	43	**1**	298	28*
chicken, McDonald's Crispy Chicken sand w/mayo	**1 oz**	65	**1**	504	24*
chicken, McDonald's Crispy Chicken sand w/o mayo	**1 oz**	55	**1**	398	24*

chicken, McDonald's McNuggets	**1 oz**	75	**6 pieces**	253	15*
chicken, Taco Bell Burrito Supreme w/chicken	**1 oz**	51	**1**	444	24*
chicken, Taco Bell soft taco w/chicken	**1 oz**	57	**1**	200	14*
chicken, Wendy's Chicken Nuggets	**1 oz**	95	**5 pieces**	250	12*
chicken, Wendy's Homestyle Chicken Fillet Sand	**1 oz**	61	**1**	492	32*
chicken, Wendy's Ultimate Chicken Grill Sandwich	**1 oz**	51	**1**	403	33*
chips, cheese flavored puffs or twists, corn based	**1 oz**	158	**6 oz**	948	10
chips, cheese flvrd puffs or twists, corn based, lowfat	**1 oz**	122	**6 oz**	732	14
chips, corn based, extruded, barbecue flavor	**1 oz**	148	**6 oz**	888	12
chips, corn based, extruded, plain	**1 oz**	147	**6 oz**	882	10
chips, potato, barbecue flavor	**1 oz**	139	**6 oz**	834	13
chips, potato, plain, salted	**1 oz**	155	**6 oz**	931	11
chips, potato, reduced fat	**1 oz**	134	**6 oz**	804	12
chips, potato, reduced fat, no salt	**1 oz**	138	**6 oz**	828	12
chips, potato, restructured, baked	**1 oz**	133	**6 oz**	798	9
chips, potato, sour cream & onion flavor	**1 oz**	151	**6 oz**	906	14
chips, taco, plain	**1 oz**	141	**6 oz**	846	13
chips, tortilla, lowfat, unsalted	**1 oz**	118	**6 oz**	708	19
chips, tortilla, nacho flavor	**1 oz**	144	**6 oz**	864	14
chips, tortilla, nacho flavor, reduced fat	**1 oz**	126	**6 oz**	756	15
chips, tortilla, taco flavor	**1 oz**	136	**6 oz**	816	13
chips, tortilla, white corn, plain	**1 oz**	138	**6 oz**	828	13
cinnamon roll, McDonald's, warm	**1 oz**	113	**3.7 oz**	418	8
cinnamon roll, McDonald's, warm deluxe	**1 oz**	104	**5.7 oz**	595	9
cinnamon roll, or sweet roll, w/raisins, commercial	**1 oz**	105	**83 g**	309	5
cinnamon roll, refrigerated dough, w/frosting	**1 oz**	94	**30 g**	100	2
cookies, brownies, commercially prepared	**1 oz**	115	**2 3/4"sq**	227	3

cookies, butter	**1 oz**	132	**5g cke**	23	<.5
cookies, chocolate chip, fast foods	**1 oz**	120	**55g box**	233	3
cookies, chocolate chip, McDonald's	**1 oz**	136	**2 oz cke**	269	3
cookies, chocolate chip, regular	**1 oz**	139	**14g cke**	68	1
cookies, chocolate, sandwich, crème filling	**1 oz**	132	**10g cke**	47	1
cookies, chocolate, sandwich, crème filling, dietary	**1 oz**	131	**10g cke**	46	<.5
cookies, chocolate, sandwich, extra crème filling	**1 oz**	141	**13g cke**	65	1
cookies, coconut macaroons	**1 oz**	115	**24g cke**	97	1
cookies, fig bars	**1 oz**	99	**16g cke**	56	1
cookies, ginger snaps	**1 oz**	118	**7g cke**	29	2
cookies, graham crackers, plain, honey, cinnamon	**1 oz**	120	**4 sq crkr**	59	1
cookies, lady fingers	**1 oz**	103	**11g cke**	40	1
cookies, marshmallow pie, chocolate coated	**1 oz**	119	**39g pie**	164	2
cookies, molasses	**1 oz**	122	**32g cke**	138	2
cookies, oatmeal, regular	**1 oz**	128	**18g cke**	81	1
cookies, peanut butter, regular	**1 oz**	135	**15g cke**	72	1
cookies, shortbread, plain	**1 oz**	142	**8g cke**	40	<.5
cookies, sugar wafers, w/crème filling	**1 oz**	145	**9g wafer**	46	<.5
cookies, sugar, regular	**1 oz**	136	**15g cke**	72	1
cookies, vanilla sandwich, w/crème filling	**1 oz**	237	**10g cke**	48	<.5
cookies, vanilla wafers	**1 oz**	125	**4g cke**	18	<.5
crackers, cheese, regular	**1 oz**	143	**1" sq**	5	<.5
crackers, cheese, sandwich-type, cheese filling	**1 oz**	139	**1sndwch**	32	<1
crackers, cheese, sandwich-type, peanut btr filling	**1 oz**	141	**1 sndwch**	32	1
crackers, graham, plain, honey, cinnamon	**1 oz**	120	**4 sq crkr**	59	1
crackers, matzo, plain	**1 oz**	112	**28g crkr**	111	3
crackers, melba toast, plain	**1 oz**	111	**5g piece**	20	1

crackers, rye, crispbread	**1 oz**	104	**10g crkr**	37	1
crackers, rye, wafers, plain	**1 oz**	95	**11g crkr**	37	1
crackers, saltine (includes oyster, soda, soup)	**1 oz**	121	**6g crkr**	26	1
crackers, standard, snack-type, regular	**1 oz**	142	**4g crkr**	20	<.5
crackers, standard, snack-type, w/cheese filling	**1 oz**	135	**7g crkr**	33	1
crackers, sandard, snack-type, w/ peanut butter fill	**1 oz**	140	**7g crkr**	35	1
crackers, wheat, regular	**1 oz**	134	**2g crkr**	9	<.5
crackers, whole wheat	**1 oz**	126	**4g crkr**	18	1
croissant, w/egg & cheese	**1 oz**	82	**1**	368	13*
croissant, w/egg, cheese, & bacon	**1 oz**	91	**1**	413	16*
croissant, w/egg, cheese, & ham	**1 oz**	88	**1**	474	19*
croissant, w/egg, cheese, & sausage	**1 oz**	93	**1**	523	20*

D

danish pastry, cheese	**1 oz**	110	**91 g**	353	6
danish pastry, cinnamon	**1 oz**	113	**88 g**	349	5
danish pastry, fruit	**1 oz**	101	**94 g**	334	5
Deluxe Breakfast, McDonald's	**1 oz**	79	**1**	1219	33*
doughnuts, cake, chocolate, glazed	**1 oz**	116	**3 3/4"d**	250	3
doughnuts, cake-type, plain	**1 oz**	119	**3 1/4"d**	198	2
doughnuts, cake-type, sugared or glazed	**1 oz**	121	**3" diam**	192	2
doughnuts, raised, glazed, yeast-leavened	**1 oz**	114	**2 oz med**	228	4
doughnuts, yeast-leavened, crème filling	**1 oz**	102	**3 oz oval**	306	5
doughnuts, yeast-leavened, jelly filling	**1 oz**	96	**3 oz**	288	5

E

éclair, custard filled w/chocolate glaze (&crème puff)	**1 oz**	74	**3 oz**	222	5
egg & cheese sandwich	**1 oz**	66	**1**	340	16*
Egg & Sausage McMuffin, McDonald's	**1 oz**	77	**1**	446	21*

Egg McMuffin, McDonald's	**1 oz**	60	**1**	290	18*
egg, ham, & cheese sandwich	**1 oz**	69	**1**	347	20*
eggs scrambled, McDonald's	**1 oz**	52	**2 eggs**	184	15*

F

fish fillet sandwich w/tartar sauce	**1 oz**	77	**1**	431	21*
fish fillet sandwich w/tartar sauce & cheese	**1 oz**	81	**1**	523	21*
frankfurter, beef	**1 oz**	94	**1 57g**	188	6*
frankfurter, beef & pork, low fat	**1 oz**	44	**1 57g**	88	6*
frankfurter, chicken	**1 oz**	64	**1 45g**	102	6*
frankfurter, meat	**1 oz**	82	**1 52g**	151	5*
frankfurter, meatless	**1 oz**	66	**1 70g**	163	14*
frankfurter, Oscar Mayer wieners, beef	**1 oz**	93	**1 45g**	147	5*
frankfurter, Oscar Mayer wieners, beef, fat free	**1 oz**	22	**1 50g**	39	7*
frankfurter, Oscar Mayer wieners, pork, turkey, beef	**1 oz**	55	**1 57g**	111	7*
frankfurter, pork	**1 oz**	76	**76g link**	204	10*
french fries, Burger King, king size	**1 oz**	94	**1**	642	7
french fries, Burger King, large	**1 oz**	94	**1**	530	6
french fries, Burger King, medium	**1 oz**	94	**1**	387	4
french fries, Burger King, small	**1 oz**	94	**1**	245	3
french fries, McDonald's, large	**1 oz**	87	**1**	522	6
french fries, McDonald's, medium	**1 oz**	87	**1**	350	4
french fries, McDonald's, small	**1 oz**	87	**1**	227	3
french fries, Wendy's, biggie	**1 oz**	90	**1**	507	6
french fries, Wendy's, great biggie	**1 oz**	90	**1**	606	7
french fries, Wendy's, medium	**1 oz**	90	**1**	453	6
french toast, w/butter	**1 oz**	75	**2 slices**	356	10
frozen novelties, vanilla ice cream w/choc coating	**1 oz**	94	**1 bar**	166	2*

G

gravy, beef, canned	**1/4 C**	30	**1 C**	123	6
gravy, chicken, canned	**1/4 C**	47	**1 C**	188	5
gravy, turkey, canned	**1/4 C**	30	**1 C**	121	6

H

ham & cheese sandwich	**1 oz**	68	**1**	352	21*
hamburger, Burger King	**1 oz**	78	**1**	333	17*
hamburger, large, double patty, w/condiments & veg	**1 oz**	68	**1**	540	34*
hamburger, large, single patty, w/condiments	**1 oz**	70	**1**	427	23*
hamburger, McDonald's	**1 oz**	71	**1**	265	13*
hamburger, regular, double patty, w/condiments	**1 oz**	76	**1**	576	32*
hamburger, regular, single patty, plain	**1 oz**	86	**1**	274	12*
hamburger, regular, single patty, w/condiments	**1 oz**	73	**1**	272	12*
hamburger, regular, single patty, w/cond & veg	**1 oz**	72	**1**	279	13*
hamburger, regular, triple patty, w/condiments	**1 oz**	76	**1**	692	50*
hamburger, Wendy's Classic single hamburger	**1 oz**	60	**1**	464	28*
hash browns, McDonald's	**1 oz**	73	**1**	136	1

I J K L M

liverwurst, pork	**1 oz**	92	**16g sl**	59	3*

N

Nachos Supreme, Taco Bell	**1 oz**	70	**1 195g**	480	15*
Nachos, Taco Bell	**1 oz**	104	**1 99g**	362	5*

O

onion rings, breaded & fried	**1 oz**	94	**8 to 9**	276	4

P

pancakes, w/butter & syrup	**1 oz**	64	**2 cakes**	520	8
pickle & pimiento loaf	**1 oz**	64	**38g sl**	86	4*

pie, apple, commercially prepared	1 oz	67	4 oz	268	2
pie, blueberry, commercially prepared	1 oz	66	4 oz	264	2
pie, cherry, commercially prepared	1 oz	74	4 oz	296	2
pie, chocolate crème, commercially prepared	1 oz	86	4 oz	344	3
pie, coconut crème, commercially prepared	1 oz	84	4 oz	336	2
pie, crust, standard type, from recipe, baked	1 oz	149	9" whole	949	12
pie, fried pie, fruit	1 oz	90	5"x3 3/4"	404	4
pie, fried pie, lemon	1 oz	90	5"x3 3/4"	404	4
pie, McDonald's baked apple pie	1 oz	92	1 pie	249	2
pie, pecan, commercially prepared	1 oz	113	4 oz	452	5
pie, pumpkin, commercially prepared	1 oz	60	4 oz	240	4
pizza, 14", cheese, regular crust	1 oz	75	1 whole	2389	108*
pizza, 14", cheese, thick crust	1 oz	77	1 whole	2655	117*
pizza, 14", cheese, thin crust	1 oz	86	1 whole	1906	89*
pizza, 14", meat & vegetable, regular crust	1 oz	69	1 whole	2850	129*
pizza, 14", pepperoni, regular crust	1 oz	78	1 whole	2647	118*
pizza, 14", pepperoni, thick crust	1 oz	81	1 whole	2826	124*
potato wedges, from frozen	1 oz	35	10 oz	350	6
pudding, instant, chocolate, prepared w/2% milk	1/2 C	155	1 C	310	9*
pudding, instant, chocolate, prepared w/whole milk	1/2 C	326	1 C	652	9*

Q R S

salami, cooked, beef	1 oz	73	26g sl	67	3*
salami, cooked, beef & pork	1 oz	71	23g sl	58	3*
salami, dry or hard, pork	1 oz	115	10g sl	41	2*
sausage, beef, cured, smoked	1 oz	88	43g saus	134	6*
sausage, Italian, pork, cooked	1 oz	98	83g link	286	16*
sausage, Polish, pork	1 oz	92	227g	740	32*

sausage, thuringer, summer, beef & pork	**1 oz**	103	**56g sl**	203	10*
shake, chocolate, McDonald's, triple thick, large	**1 oz**	46	**1 32 oz**	1162	26*
shake, chocolate, McDonald's, triple thick, medium	**1 oz**	46	**1 21 oz**	771	17*
shake, chocolate, McDonald's, triple thick, small	**1 oz**	46	**1 16 oz**	580	13*
shake, strawberry, McDonald's, triple thick, large	**1 oz**	45	**1 32 oz**	1119	25*
shake, strawberry, McDonald's, triple thick, medium	**1 oz**	45	**1 21 oz**	741	16*
shake, strawberry, McDonald's, triple thick, small	**1 oz**	45	**1 16 oz**	559	12*
shake, vanilla, Burger King, medium	**1 oz**	42	**1 16 oz**	667	13*
shake, vanilla, Burger King, small	**1 oz**	42	**1 12 oz**	501	10*
shake, vanilla, McDonald's, triple thick, large	**1 oz**	35	**1 32 oz**	1104	25*
shake, vanilla, McDonald's, triple thick, medium	**1 oz**	35	**1 21 oz**	733	16*
shake, vanilla, McDonald's, triple thick, small	**1 oz**	35	**1 16 oz**	552	12*

T U V W X Y Z

taco salad	**1 oz**	40	**1.5 C**	279	13
taco salad, Taco Bell	**1 oz**	48	**1 533g**	906	35*
taco, large	**1 oz**	61	**1 263g**	568	32*
taco, original, w/beef, Taco Bell	**1 oz**	67	**1 78g**	184	8*
taco, small	**1 oz**	61	**1 171g**	369	21*
taco, soft, w/beef, Taco Bell	**1 oz**	62	**1 99g**	217	12*
taco, soft, w/chicken, Taco Bell	**1 oz**	57	**1 99g**	200	14*
taco, soft, w/steak, Taco Bell	**1 oz**	64	**1 127g**	286	15*

www.ingramcontent.com/pod-product-compliance
Lightning Source LLC
Chambersburg PA
CBHW080449290526
45791CB00008BA/2656